Contents

Introduction

This booklet aims to help you understand more about self-harm and what to do if you are worried about yourself or someone else. It explains what self-harm is, what to do if you or someone you know is self-harming, and how to get help.

Self-harm is very common and affects more people than you might think.

'10% of young people self-harm'

This means that it's likely that at least two young people in every secondary school classroom have self-harmed at some time. If you are self-harming, you are not alone – lots of information and support are available.

Remember, self-harm isn't a suicide attempt or a cry for attention. However, it can be a way for some people to cope with overwhelming and distressing thoughts or feelings. Self-harm should be taken seriously, whatever the reason behind it.

It is possible to live without self-harm. It is important to know that you won't always feel the way you do now.

With the right help and support most people who self-harm can and do fully recover.

What is self-harm?

Self-harm describes any behaviour where someone causes harm to themselves, usually as a way to help cope with difficult or distressing thoughts and feelings. It most frequently takes the form of cutting, burning or non-lethal overdoses. However, it can also be any behaviour that causes injury – no matter how minor, or high-risk behaviours.

Basically, any behaviour that that causes harm or injury to someone as a way to deal with difficult emotions can be seen as self-harm.

The self-harm cycle

Self-harm usually starts as a way to relieve the build-up of pressure from distressing thoughts and feelings. This might give temporary relief from the emotional pain the person is feeling. It's important to know that this relief is only temporary because the underlying reasons still remain. Soon after, feelings of guilt and shame might follow, which can continue the cycle.

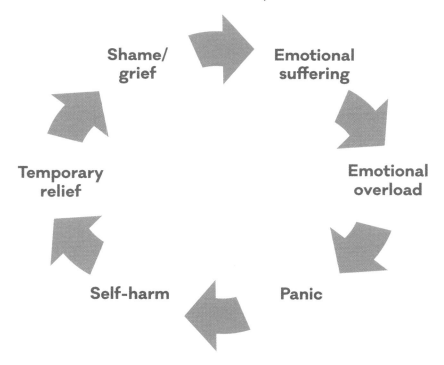

Because there may be some temporary relief at the start, self-harm can become someone's normal way of dealing with life's difficulties. This means that it is important to talk to someone as early as possible to get the right support and help. Learning new coping strategies to deal with these difficulties can make it easier to break the cycle of self-harm in the long term.

Who does it?

There is no such thing as a typical young person who self-harms. **Self-harm is something that can affect anyone**. It's believed that around 10% of young people self-harm, but it could be as high as 20%. If you self-harm, there are a lot of people who also know what you're going through.

'Most young people reported that they started to hurt themselves around the age of 12.'

While it is true that anyone can be affected by self-harm, some people are more likely to self-harm than others because of things that have happened in their lives - where they live, things that are happening with friends, family or at school, or a combination of these. This means that some people are more at risk of self-harm than others.

Some factors that might make someone more at risk are:

- Experience of a mental health disorder. This might include depression, anxiety, borderline personality disorder, and eating disorders.
- Being a young person who is not under the care of their parents, or young people who have left a care home.
- Being part of the LGBT community.
- Having been bereaved by suicide.

It is important to remember that although these are risk factors that can make someone more likely to self-harm, having any of these does not mean someone will self-harm. Similarly, someone who self-harms might not experience any of these. Anyone can be affected.

Why do people self-harm?

Everyone has different things that cause stress and worry them. Some people can manage these troubles by talking to friends and family, while others may find these difficulties overwhelming. When we don't express our emotions and talk about the things that make us distressed, angry or upset, the pressure can build up and become unbearable. Some people turn this in on themselves and use their bodies as a way to express the thoughts and feelings they can't say aloud. People often harm themselves when this all gets too much. If you self-harm, you might find that when you feel angry, distressed, worried or depressed, you feel the urge to hurt yourself even more.

Someone's reason to self-harm can be very different from other people who self-harm. Some of the reasons that young people report as triggers or reasons that lead them to self-harm include:

- difficulties at home
- arguments or problems with friends
- school pressures
- bullying
- depression
- anxiety
- low self-esteem
- transitions and changes, such as changing schools
- alcohol and drug use.

When a few of these issues come together they can quickly feel overwhelming and become too much for one person to deal with. As one young person said, many people self-harm to *'get out the hurt, anger and pain'* caused by pressures in their lives. They hurt themselves because they didn't know what else to do and didn't feel like they had any other options. Talking to someone you trust or a healthcare professional can help you find other options for coping with the emotional pain you are feeling.

If you are experiencing difficult issues in your life, there is support available. Please see the 'Further help, support and information?' section of this booklet (pages 34-35).

Breaking down the myths

There are lots of myths attached to self-harm. This isn't surprising – myths and misunderstandings often arise when a problem like self-harm is poorly understood. Negative stereotypes can be powerful. They need to be challenged because they stop people talking about their issues and asking for help. These myths also mean that professionals, family and friends can misunderstand people who self-harm.

MYTH: 'Self-harm is attention-seeking'

One of the most common stereotypes is that self-harm is about 'attention seeking'. This is not the case. Many people who self-harm don't talk to anyone about what they are going through for a long time and it can be very hard for them to find enough courage to ask for help.

MYTH: 'Self-harm is a goth thing'

Self-harm has been stereotyped to be seen as part of youth subcultures such as "goth" or "emo". While there is some research suggesting a link, there is no conclusive evidence of this with little or no evidence supporting the belief that self-harm is part of any particular young person subculture.

MYTH: 'Only girls self-harm'

It is often assumed that girls are more likely than boys to self-harm, however it isn't clear if this is true. Boys and girls may engage with different self-harming behaviours or have different reasons for hurting themselves, but this doesn't make it any less serious.

MYTH: 'People who self-harm must enjoy it'

Some people believe that people who self-harm take pleasure in the pain or risk associated in the behaviour. There is no evidence that people who self-harm feel pain differently than anyone else. The harming behaviour often causes people great pain. For some, being depressed has left them numb and they want to feel anything to remind them they are alive, even if it hurts. Others have described this pain as punishment.

MYTH: 'People who self-harm are suicidal'

Self-harm is sometimes viewed as a suicide attempt by people who don't understand it. For many people self-harm is about trying to cope with difficult feelings and circumstances. Some people have described it as a way of staying alive and surviving these difficulties. However, some people who self-harm can feel suicidal and might attempt to take their own life, which is why it must always be taken seriously.

'People often link self-harm to suicide but for me it was something very different; it was my alternative to suicide, my way of coping even though sometimes I wished that my world would end.'

Getting help

Should I tell someone?

Yes. Talking to someone is often the first step to getting out of the cycle.

It isn't an easy thing to do and you might find it difficult to talk about your self-harm and the reasons behind it. This is normal - lots of young people who self-harm find asking for help very difficult. But it is an important step towards recovery and feeling better.

'Telling someone about your self-harm shows strength and courage; it can often be a huge relief to be able to let go of such a secret, or at least share it.'

Don't be afraid to ask for help whenever and however you need to. Talking about your feelings isn't a sign of weakness. It shows that you are taking charge of your well-being and doing what you need to stay healthy. It isn't always easy to express how you are feeling. If you can't think of one word to describe a feeling, use as many as you need to illustrate how you feel.

Talking can be a way of coping with a problem you've been carrying around in your head for a while. Feeling listened to can help you feel more supported. And it works both ways: if you open up it might encourage others to do the same.

Who can I talk to?

There are lots of people you can talk to about what you are going through. It is important to tell someone you trust and feel comfortable with, as they will be able to help and support you. Young people told us that they have been able to talk to:

- friends
- family
- someone at school, such as a trusted teacher, school nurse or pastoral care staff
- a youth worker
- their GP or healthcare professionals such as a counsellor or nurse
- charities and helplines (some of which are listed on pages 32-33).

There are no rules about how you should tell someone. The most important thing is that you feel comfortable and trust the person you decide to tell. Set time aside to talk to them. Remember you can set the pace and it is up to you how much you want to tell them.

If you find speaking about it too difficult, you can tell someone in writing or in an email. You can even ask a friend to speak to a trusted adult on your behalf. Let them know you need help with how you are feeling. There is no need to give details about how you have harmed yourself and you don't need to talk about things you feel uncomfortable talking about. Try to focus on the thoughts and feelings behind your self-harm rather than the behaviours.

If you decide to talk to a GP or other health professional, you can take a friend or family member with you to support you.

'Sometimes after telling someone you may feel worse. That's normal. But remember that once you get over this hurdle there is support and help available.'

If you're worried that when you tell someone they won't understand, or if you have experienced this, try giving them a copy of this booklet or suggest they talk to an expert in the field to try to understand more about self-harm.

Remember that health professionals, GPs and teachers are familiar with this issue and are there to help.

Don't let the fear of a bad reaction put you off seeking the help you need and deserve. As hard as it is to tell someone, sharing will take the pressure off you and help you get the right support and help available.

What help is available for me?

There are lots of support services and treatments available when you feel ready to seek help. If you seek help from your GP, it is likely they will offer you counselling, where a professional will listen and help you to work on solutions and strategies to cope with the problems you are dealing with.

Talking therapies such as cognitive behavioural therapy (CBT) focus on building coping strategies and problem-solving skills and have been found to be very effective in helping to reduce self-harm.

Other forms of counselling, like psychodynamic therapy, for instance, will help you to identify the problems that are causing you distress and leading you to self-harm. It is important that you talk to your GP or a trusted health professional who will help decide the best treatment option for you.

There are also a number of charities and self-help groups throughout the UK that can support you through this experience. People who have self-harmed have said that it can be helpful to hear from other young people who have experienced self-harm. More information about these sources of support is available at the end of this booklet.

'I feel a lot more confident. I've learned to be more open about my feelings and been able to move on. I felt that, without them knowing, I was being held back. I've been able to come out of myself and explain what I do, and make sense of it, not keep having to lie and cover up what I did. I no longer feel ashamed as I know people are supporting me.'

Recovery

It's important to remember that you won't always feel the way you do now. The problems that are causing you to self-harm can, with help and support, become more manageable over time or even go away. Things can and do get better!

'Take time and be patient with yourself. Recovery doesn't happen overnight - it can be a slow process. Start to learn how to care for yourself.'

Young people who have recovered from self-harm say that changes over time and changes in circumstances in life (for example moving home, changing schools, finishing exams, going to university, changing jobs or changed financial circumstances) helped them to recover. Once one or two of the main factors that were causing them to self-harm (such as their family situation, or bullying at school) were removed, they felt they didn't have to use self-harm as a coping strategy.

Others explained that recovery was about finding new coping strategies and more helpful ways of dealing with emotions or distress. This is also an important factor towards recovery from self-harm.

'It dawned on me that continually harming myself was not allowing me to grow; it was just proving that I was still here and I could feel. But wasn't letting me push things forward, and unless I stopped doing that, I would be in the same situation forever.'

How can I stop harming myself?

Asking for help and having support is very important if you are trying to stop self-harming. It is important that you do this when you feel ready to talk about it. It doesn't matter who you talk to, as long as it's someone you trust and feel comfortable with. Talking to someone is what is important. You don't have to feel that you need to deal with this on your own. For young people used to carrying burdens on their own, it can be hard to receive support. Part of recovery is trusting people enough to let them help you.

Talking to someone you trust can help you discover why you self-harm and help to find new ways to cope with difficulties. Finding out what makes you happy, sad, angry, isolated, vulnerable or strong can help you develop other ways of dealing with these feelings. Counselling is a good way of exploring these thoughts and feelings and is available through your GP.

Other young people who have self-harmed have found 'distraction techniques' to be a very useful strategy to reduce or stop self-harming. These techniques find a release for the emotional pressure you feel without the need to harm.

'If you feel the need to harm yourself, try to give yourself a goal of getting through the next ten minutes without doing so.'

Distraction techniques

When you feel the urge to self-harm, distraction techniques can be a useful way to 'ride the wave' of emotion and overcome the urge to harm yourself.

Young people shared their most helpful ones with us:

- Write down thoughts and feelings that are distressing you; crumple the page up, rip it apart and throw them out as a way to let go of that thought.
- Get some play-dough: stretch it or squeeze it to relieve tension.
- Hit a pillow or cushion to vent your anger and frustration.
- Have a good scream into a pillow or cushion.
- Take a minute and breathe or meditate.
- Go for a walk to take yourself away from triggers. Being in a public place gives you the time and space to reduce the urge to hurt yourself.
- Make lots of noise, either with a musical instrument or just banging on pots and pans.
- Scribble on a large piece of paper with a red crayon or pen.
- Call a friend or family member and talk to them. This doesn't have to be about self-harm.
- Do something creative: make a collage of colours to represent your mood or to remind you of your favourite things.
- Listen to music you like or watch a film you enjoy.

- Go online and look at self-help websites.
- Talk to someone about what is triggering you or seek help from a professional.

'I've tried so many distraction techniques – from writing down my thoughts, hitting a pillow, listening to music, writing down pros and cons. But the most helpful to my recovery was the five minutes rule, where if you feel like you want to self-harm, you wait for five minutes before you do it, then see if you can go another five minutes, and so on till eventually the feeling that you need to is over.'

Tips for looking after yourself

Keeping safe

Self-harm is not a positive way to deal with things. However if you are self-harming it can be difficult to stop, especially when you feel distressed or upset. If you don't feel you can stop right now, it is important that you do keep yourself safe.

Wounds and injuries of any type can be dangerous and carry the risk of infection, which can be serious, so they need to be looked after. If you have serious injury, feel unwell or feel that you are going into shock (fast breathing, racing heart, feeling faint or panicked) you should seek help immediately. If you find yourself in this situation, find a trusted adult or friend who can get you the medical attention you need. This doesn't mean you have to discuss your self-harm with them (although it may help); it is about allowing someone to support you medically in a moment of crisis.

Make a 'safe box'

You can create a safe box to help you through times when you feel overwhelmed by emotion and have the urge to harm yourself. Fill it with things that make you happy and calm, to help you to get through this feeling. Some suggestions: activities such as crosswords, your favourite book, CD or movie. You could also include a list of things to do that make you calm when you are feeling triggered.

Talk to someone

When you are feeling overwhelmed, talk to a friend, family member or trusted adult. Let them know what you are thinking. This can help relieve the pressure that you are feeling. Make a list of people you can talk to at these times and keep it somewhere safe. Knowing who you can talk to in times of crisis at 3am, weekends or when you are at school can make it easier to ask for help when you need it. Add these to your safe box. This will remind you that you are not alone and there are people you can talk to when you need to.

Avoid alcohol and drugs

We often drink alcohol or take drugs to change our mood or to avoid our feelings. Some people drink to deal with fear or loneliness, but like self-harm the effect is only temporary and can end up making you feel worse. Alcohol is a depressant, which means it slows down brain activity. This changes how you think and feel, so can increase feelings of anxiety and depression. When it wears off you can end up feeling worse because of the effects it has on your brain and your body.

Drinking alcohol or taking drugs can leave you feeling depressed or anxious, and can lower your inhibitions physically, which can lead you back to harming yourself. Visit www.drinkaware.co.uk for more information.

Do something you enjoy

Remember that there is more to you than self-harm. Do things that remind you of this and make you happy. Maybe this is a sport, or a hobby you like doing such as writing.

Doing things that you enjoy and makes you feel happy, helps you look after your mental health. It helps to improve your self-esteem and can help you remember that you are important and have value.

Don't be too hard on yourself

Many young people who self-harm can be perfectionists and high achievers. You might put pressure on yourself to do things in a certain way, or feel that nothing you do is good enough.

Try to not be so hard on yourself about not getting things perfect. Recovery is about knowing that it is okay for your work or performance to be 'good enough'.

'Many people stop hurting themselves when the time is right for them. Everyone is different and if they feel the need to self-harm at the moment, they shouldn't feel guilty about it – it is a way of surviving, and doing it now does NOT mean that they will need to do it forever. It is a huge step towards stopping when they begin to talk about it, because it means that they are starting to think about what might take its place eventually.'

I am worried about someone else

If you are worried that someone you know is self-harming, it is important to know what to look out for and what to do. Below is some information to help you.

Signs to look out for

It can be difficult to tell whether someone is self-harming. Here are some signs that might suggest someone could be self-harming:

- Withdrawal or isolation from everyday life.
- Signs of depression such as low mood, tearfulness or a lack of motivation or interest in anything.
- Changes in mood.
- Changes in eating/sleeping habits.
- Changes in activity and mood, e.g. more aggressive than usual.
- Talking about self-harming or suicide.
- Abusing drugs or alcohol.
- Expressing feelings of failure, uselessness or loss of hope.
- Risk taking behaviour (substance misuse, unprotected sexual acts).
- Signs of low self-esteem such as blaming themselves for any problems or saying they are not good enough.

- Unexplained cuts, bruises or marks.
- Covering up all the time, when in hot weather.
- Being quieter than usual.
- Lacking energy.

It is important to know that these may be a sign of other things and don't always mean someone is self-harming. Also, there may be **no** warning signs at all. It is therefore important that if you suspect someone you know is self-harming, that you ask them openly and honestly.

What to do if you are worried about someone

If you are worried that someone you know is self-harming, it can be difficult to know what to do. When you are aware there is an issue, it is important that you do not wait. Waiting and hoping they will come to you for help might lose valuable time in getting them the best support and treatment to help them.

Be mindful that they might not feel ready or able to talk about their self-harm. Let them lead the discussion at their own pace and don't put pressure on them to tell you details that they aren't ready to talk about. It takes a lot of trust and courage to open up about self-harm. You might be the first person they have been able to talk to about this.

Some tips for talking to someone about self-harm:

- Set plenty of time aside to talk to them where you will be free from interruption. If you don't have time at that particular moment, make sure to put time later in the day when you can listen to them.

- If possible, remove distractions such as computers and phones being on. This will allow you to give your full attention, letting them know you are there to listen to and support them.

- Acknowledge how difficult it might be to open up about their self-harm but don't focus on or encourage them to tell you details about specific injuries or behaviours. Instead talk about how they are feeling and what they are going through.

- Try not to react shocked or disgusted. This can be hard as it can be difficult to understand why someone would harm themselves, but negative reactions can hurt the other person and may put them off talking to you.

- Know your limits. The person who has experienced self-harm might tell you to keep it a secret and not to tell anyone else. If you believe they are in immediate danger or have injuries that need medical attention, you need to take action to make sure they are safe.

- Reassure them that you are there for them and that there are lots of sources of support available to them. You might not understand what they are going through or why they do it but remind them you are there for them regardless.

- Avoid giving ultimatums; for example 'stop or else...' as these rarely work, and may drive behaviours underground. Furthermore, this may stop them talking to you and you might not get the chance to discuss the topic again.

- Offer them help in seeking professional support and provide information on ways to do this. You might want to offer to go the GP with them, or help them talk to a trusted adult or family member. Try not to take control and allow them to make decisions.

- Be positive and let them know that things will get better and recovery is possible !

Key points:

- make time
- listen
- be open and honest
- don't judge
- offer support
- remember the person behind the behaviour.

If it is a family member or close friend you are concerned about, they might not want to talk to you. Try not to take this personally: telling someone you love about self-harm can be difficult as you are close to them and they might be worried they are hurting you.

Whether you approach someone you are worried about, or someone opens up to you about their self-harm, it is important that you respond in a non-judgemental, caring and respectful way. This can be hard when you see that someone is in distress, and it can be difficult to understand why someone would hurt themselves, however you should try to see the person and reasons they have harmed themselves rather than focusing on the behaviours.

Further help, information and support

If you are worried about the immediate well-being of yourself or someone else you should call 999 or go straight to A & E. For non-emergency help you should talk to your GP or contact 111 or NHS Direct on 08454647.

You can also get more information or support through the websites below:

SelfHarm.co.uk – www.selfharm.co.uk

selfharmUK is a project dedicated to supporting young people impacted by self-harm, providing a safe space to talk, ask any questions and be honest about what's going on in your life. These pages will tell you a bit about us as well as pointing you in the right direction if you need to contact us or find out more about our policies and procedures.

Young Minds - www.youngminds.org.uk

YoungMinds is the UK's leading charity committed to improving the emotional wellbeing and mental health of children and young people. Driven by their experiences we campaign, research and influence policy and practice.

Some websites that have been recommended to us by young people include:

- www.lifesigns.org.uk
- www.childline.org.uk
- www.selfharm.org.uk
- www.youngminds.org.uk
- www.b-eat.co.uk
- www.samaritans.org.uk
- www.harmless.org.uk

Some telephone helplines offer specialist advice on self-harm, others operate only as a 'friendly listening ear' – something many young people have said they value, particularly when they feel they have no-one else that they can turn to. Again, it's important that information about reputable phone lines is widely available to young people. Helpful telephone numbers include:

- ChildLine – 0800 1111
- Samaritans – 08457 90 90 90
- Family Lives – 0808 800 2222
- Young Minds – 0808 802 5544
- Get Connected – 0808 808 4994

Notes

Notes

Notes